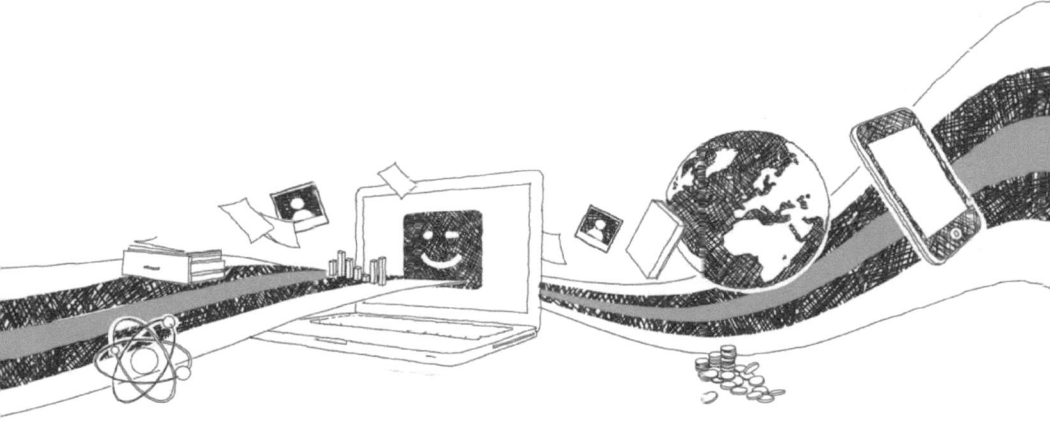
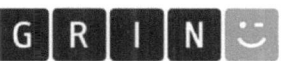

Bibliographic information published by the German National Library:

The German National Library lists this publication in the National Bibliography; detailed bibliographic data are available on the Internet at http://dnb.dnb.de .

Imprint:

Copyright © 2010 GRIN Verlag, Open Publishing GmbH
Print and binding: Books on Demand GmbH, Norderstedt Germany
ISBN: 9783640976737

This book at GRIN:

http://www.grin.com/en/e-book/176302/12-step-addiction-treatment

Hans Durrer

12-Step Addiction Treatment

Does AA Work?

GRIN Publishing

GRIN - Your knowledge has value

Since its foundation in 1998, GRIN has specialized in publishing academic texts by students, college teachers and other academics as e-book and printed book. The website www.grin.com is an ideal platform for presenting term papers, final papers, scientific essays, dissertations and specialist books.

Visit us on the internet:

http://www.grin.com/

http://www.facebook.com/grincom

http://www.twitter.com/grin_com

Hans Durrer

12-Step Addiction Treatment

Does AA Work?

Content

ABSTRACT

A comprehensive literature review was undertaken that was compared to the author's own AA-experience in various cultures. The search was neither restricted to a specific time period nor were language restrictions employed. Studies published in peer-reviewed, academic journals as well as books and websites were selected on the basis of "usefulness" in regards to the research question. After establishing what AA is, the essay examined whether AA works. It found that AA differs substantially in regards to other treatment approaches by it's "acting into thinking"-philosophy. The efficacy of AA could not be proven by employing a cause-and-effect methodology. Moreover, the complexity of human behaviour as well as the fact that AA is not practised uniformly raises many seemingly unanswerable methodological problems and it remains questionable whether AA treatment and outcomes can be measured by a cause-and-effect method. Testimonies of personal experience as well as for centuries practised human wisdom seem however to suggest that AA does work – for the ones who work the programme, that is.

1. METHODOLOGY

This study of whether AA works consists of a comprehensive literature review that was compared to the author's own AA-experience in various cultures. The search was neither restricted to a specific time period nor were language restrictions employed. The following search terms were used (both individually and in various combinations – the list is not exhaustive) in Google and Yahoo: alcohol treatment, treatment outcomes, alcohol treatment efficacy, addiction treatment effectiveness, AA success, alcohol treatment outcomes, measuring treatment, addiction therapy success, alcohol therapy success, twelve step effectiveness, twelve step efficacy, AA programme, AA promises, cause and effect proof, recovery, definition recovery, AA cult, AA religion, AA testimonials, AA statistics, personal AA experiences, addiction treatment scientific evidence.

The following databases were searched: Alcohol Concern Online Library, Drugscope database, NIDA database, Robin Room Archive, SAMHSA's National Clearinghouse for Alcohol and Drug Information, Scottish Addiction Studies Online Library, Social Science Information Gateway, Stirling University Library E-Journal Gateway, World Health Organization database.

Blogs and websites searched: Addiction Search, Alcoholic Anonymous, Alcohol Reports, Dirk Hanson's Chemical Carousel Website, Drink and Drugs News Website, Spiritual River Website, The Orange Papers, The Stanton Peele Addiction Website, Wired in to Recovery Website, Websites of Recovery Centers.

The following journals were searched: Addiction, Addiction Research & Theory, Addiction Treatment Forum, Alcohol, Alcohol and Alcoholism, Alcohol Research & Health, BMC Health Services Research, Drug and Alcohol Dependence, Drug and Alcohol Findings, Journal of Substance Abuse Treatment, The Journal of Studies on Alcohol and Drugs.

Selection criteria for studies retained: blogs and websites were mainly used in order to "get a feel" for the various ideological positions held. Otherwise there were no particular restrictions: studies published in peer-reviewed, academic journals as well as books were exclusively selected on the basis whether they were able to meaningfully contribute to the research question.

The study proceeds in the following way: In a first step, it attempts to outline what AA is before, in a second step, examining whether AA works. A third step finally discusses the findings before, in a final step, a conclusion is presented.

2. FINDINGS

2.1 WHAT IS AA?

The book "Alcoholics Anonymous" (1994), also known as the "Big Book", is considered the "basic text for our Society" (Alcoholics Anonymous 1994: i) and names as the essentials of the AA-approach "the need for moral inventory, confession of personality defects, restitution to those harmed, helpfulness to others, and the necessity of belief in and dependence upon God" (*Ibid,* vi).

The following statement is read out load at the start of AA meetings and is aimed at reminding the participants what these meetings should be all about:

Alcoholics Anonymous is a fellowship of men and women who share their experience, strength and hope with each other that they may solve their common problem and help others to recover from alcoholism. The only requirement for membership is a desire to stop drinking. There are no dues or fees for AA membership; we are self-supporting through our own contributions. AA is not allied with any sect, denomination, politics, organization or institution; does not wish to engage in any controversy, neither endorses nor opposes any causes. Our primary purpose is to stay sober and help other alcoholics to achieve sobriety" (This is A.A. 1984).

The AA programme is based on the twelve steps and the twelve traditions (see appendix). It is a spiritual programme – *"spiritus contra spiritum",* as C.G. Jung penned in a letter to Bill Wilson (Alcoholics Anonymous 1984: 384) - and explicitly states that only a Higher Power can relieve sufferers from their alcoholism.

Our description of the alcoholic, the chapter to the agnostic, and our personal adventures before and after make clear three pertinent ideas: (a) That we were alcoholic and could not manage our own lives. (b) That probably no human power could have relieved our alcoholism. (c) That God could and would if He were sought (Alcoholics Anonymous 1994: 60).

This seems to suggest that AA is a religious movement. In fact, Jacques T. (1991: 50) affirms that the twelve steps, when practised, do not differ from the dramatic conversion that Saint Paul experienced on the road to Damascus. A conversion is central to the AA programme. As William James in *The Varieties of Religious Experience*, by which Bill Wilson, one of the founders of AA, was deeply influenced, states:

... the salvation through self-despair, the dying to be truly born, of Lutheran theology, the passage into <u>nothing</u> of which Jakob Behmen writes. To get to it, a critical point must usually be passed, a corner turned within one. Something must give way, a native hardness must break down and liquefy; and this event (as well shall abundantly see

4

hereafter) is frequently sudden and automatic, and leaves on the Subject an impression that he has been wrought on by an external power (James 1994: 125).

In other words, "a new human being has to be created", as Enquist (2008: 494) noted, and added that this might meet with resistence.

There are statements by Bill Wilson that suggest that AA is a religion. For instance: "I must turn in all things to the Father of Light who presides over us all" (Alcoholics Anonymous 1994: 12). Moreover, five of the twelve steps mention God (and/or Him) explicitly and quite some meetings that I attended closed with the Lord's Prayer. In spite of that the "Big Book' clearly states: "Alcoholics Anonymous is not a religious organization" (Alcoholics Anonymous 1994: x).

Yet "... federal courts have asserted, AA is unequivocally religious.' They only looked at AA's doctrinal literature, and unhesitatingly declared what is obvious to anyone" (Trimpey 1997). And Rudy and Greil (1988: 41) opine: "A.A. is properly classified as a quasi-religion in so far as a tension between sacred and secular is crucial to its functioning."

There are dangers of distorting a treatment ideology with quasi-religious overtones, as Goethals, Broekaert and Yates (forthcoming) point out, and AA has indeed quasi-religious overtones and also cult-like elements: members who revere Bill Wilson as if he were a saint, for example, or the ones who read the Big Book as if it were written by God. As the writer Wilfrid Sheed (1995: 89) notes: "In the new world I was about to enter, the assumption was that it was always the truth you were flinching from like a vampire at high noon, and never just from cliché or, in this case, a shower of clichés, the bane of my profession". Yet AA is clearly not a cult: it has no leader, makes no financial demands, does not coerce people into the programme (with the exception of US courts) and everybody is free to leave (Bufe 1998). As the "Big Book" states: "We are not allied with any particular faith, sect or denomination, nor do we oppose anyone" (Alcoholics Anonymous 1994: iv).

To look at the AA literature is one way to approach AA, to look at the fellowship in action another. While the format of AA meetings is the same all over the world (there are all sorts of meetings, from step-meetings to discussion-meetings, open and closed ones etc.), it is the ones attending who decide how these meetings are conducted and who create the vibes (and it is often these vibes that make people stay or leave). I've heard of meetings in the Philippines, and in Italy, where, allegedly, alcohol was consumed, have participated in meetings that I've found difficult to bear in the sense that David Foster Wallace (1995) described: "So then at forty-six years of age I came here to learn to live by clichés ... To turn my will and life over to the care of clichés. One day at a time. Easy does it. First things first. Ask for help. Thy will not mine be done. It works if you work it. Grow or go. Keep coming back", and I've been to meetings where I felt profoundly helped by the stories shared. In other words, what AA do we refer to when asking whether it works?

Miller and Rollnick (2009) hold that, in the late 20th century, the 12-step model was quite at variance with original descriptions of the AA programme. "At some point, such a reinvention no longer contains and may even violate the spirit and elements that defined the original approach" (Miller and Rollnick 2009: 130). In addition, as a 36 year member of AA in 1976 penned: "There are three ways to work the program of Alcoholics Anonymous. (1) The strong, original way, proved powerfully and reliably effective over forty years. (2) A medium way – not so strong, not so safe, not so sure, not so good, but still effective. And (3) a weak way, which turns out to be really no way at all but literally a heresy, a false teaching, a twisting corruption of what the founders of Alcoholics Anonymous clearly stated the program to be" (24 Magazine 1976).

In sum: On the one hand, there seem to be as many interpretations of AA as there are AA members. On the other hand, there are the ones who appear to regard not only the „Big Book" as a sacred text but also advice like "90 meetings in 90 days" and "Get a sponsor" that cannot be found in the „Big Book". And then there are the ones like me who take from the programme what they like and leave the rest. In other words, it is questionable whether the voluntary and informal nature of AA allows for an assessment that meets scientific criteria.

2.2   DOES AA WORK?

"To share your experience, strength and hope in order to stay sober - that is basically the AA-secret formula" writes Zocker (1989: 19). The "Big Book" states:

Rarely have we seen a person fail who has thoroughly followed our path. Those who do not recover are people who cannot or will not completely give themselves to this simple program, usually men and women who are constitutionally incapable of being honest with themselves. There are such unfortunates. They are not at fault; they seem to have been born that way. They are naturally incapable of grasping and developing a manner of living which demands rigorous honesty. Their chances are less than average. There are those, too, who suffer from grave emotional and mental disorders, but many of them do recover if they have the capacity to be honest (Alcoholics Anonymous 1994: 58).

In other words, rigorous honesty is key for getting, and staying, sober: if you're honest you will recover. And if you do not recover, you simply haven't been honest. Ludwig (1989: 4) comments: "Along with other addictions, alcoholism is unique in the extent to which the individual is blamed if the treatment fails. If the alcoholic does not remain abstinent, therapists and staff presume that he is unmotivated for or unreceptive to help."

This insistence on honesty is by no means limited to Christianity – to ask whether AA is a religion means whether it is a Christian religion – but an ancient wisdom that is shared by Buddha, Socrates, Spinoza, Hegel and Marx (Fromm 1979: 7). The same applies to the hero-myth that, according to Joseph Campbell (Maher and Briggs 1989), exists in all cultures and shows "obvious parallels between the processes of addiction and recovery and the structure of the hero's tale. There are hundreds of thousands of people whose recovery stories share striking similarities to Campbell's myth of the hero" (White 2007a).

In 1955, AA claimed that of the ones who "really tried, 50% got sober at once and remained that way; 25% sobered up after some relapses, and among the remainder, those who stayed on with A.A. showed improvement" (Alcoholics Anonymous 1994: x). Yet how does one measure "really tried"?

In 1972, an anonymous writer argued in 24 Magazine (1976) "that as AA has gotten bigger and older, its effectiveness has dropped from about three in four to about two in three." In the same article it says: "two in three was in 1976 – our data shows numbers much LESS in 1997 – 1 in 15".

In 1989, Robertson (1989: 108) claimed that 60 percent of all newcomers to AA who stay for about a year will generally stay sober forever.

Such claims are however disputed. According to Peele (1998), "AA succeeds with relatively few (5% at most) of the massive numbers of alcoholics who wander through its meetings." And, as Ludwig states, only about 10 percent of all those who recover do so through AA (Ludwig 1988: 67).

Since AA "does not publish data on its participants' success rate" (Carey 2008: D1), one wonders where these figures come from. Besides, difficulties in measuring treatment success are manifold. For instance: ' The resort-and-spa private clinics generally do not allow outside researchers to verify their published success rates. The publicly supported programs spend their scarce resources on patient care, not costly studies" (Carey 2008: D1). Moreover, there are no standard guidelines in the field. "Each program has its own philosophy; so, for that matter, do individual counselors. No one knows which approach is best for which patient, because these programs rarely if ever track clients closely after they graduate" (Carey 2008: D1).

However, outcome studies have investigated the relationship between AA attendance and length of abstinence and found that AA members report greater abstinence than nonmembers and that the longer the membership in AA the greater the length of sobriety is (Le, Ingvarson and Page 1995).

Project MATCH was a study that aimed to establish what works for whom in regards to alcohol abuse and drug dependency. The hypothesis was that treatment that would adress the individual patient's needs and characteristics would surely yield better results than one which would treat all patients (with the same diagnosis) in the same manner (Project MATCH Research Group 1993). It found that treatments (Cognitive Behavioral Coping Skills, Motivational Enhancement Therapy, Twelve-Step Facilitation) didn't differ in effectiveness when applied to a heterogeneous group. Culter and Fishbain re-examined the study and pointed out that "a median of only 3% of the drinking outcome at follow-up could be attributed to treatment. However this effect appeared to be present at week one before most of the treatment had been delivered. The zero treatment dropout group showed great improvement, achieving a mean of 72 percent days abstinent at follow-up" (Culter and Fishbain 2005). Peele criticised the lack of a control group and that the effectiveness was measured by reduction in frequency and intensity of drinking while the 12-step approach is based on total abstinence (Peele 1998a)
In sum, there is little empirical evidence to support the notion of patient matching. Moreover, questions in regards to the typicality of the client sample have persisted (Velasquez, DiClemente and Addy 2000: 179).

In 1994, a treatment outcome evaluation of 65,000 patients by CATOR found that "people who complete treatment but who don't follow through with either self-help support group attendance or regular continuing professional contacts have a less than 50 percent chance of staying sober; those who follow through with both have a greater than 80 percent probability of greater sobriety" (West 1997: 146).

The most recent study on treatment effictiveness is DATOS, carried out in a decade of widespread cocaine (especially crack) use in the US and seems to prove that treatment (12-step philosophies dominated) works. "A year after teatment, drug use, illegal activities and psychological stress had fallen by about 50%" (Franey and Ashton 2002: 5). In regards to treatment modalities, the study found that: "Delivered with sufficient quality, they are *all* effective" (Franey and Ashton 2002: 18).

Yet, how can one know whether people who attend AA meetings are really alcoholics (I know of people who, admittedly, did not have alcohol problems but simply liked the vibes at meetings) or, if they were, would have not become sober naturally due to life stages and/or environmental factors? (Vaillant 1983; Peele 1995). As Yates (1997: 30) points out:

What limits outcome monitoring is that even the most loyal client will probably only spend a tiny part of their life visiting drug or alcohol services. A lot of other things will be going on in their lives which will almost certainly have a much bigger effect on their health and behaviour. These outside forces may be stronger at some times than at others ... Put simply, there is no way of proving whether changes identified in service users use of drugs/drink etc. have to do with their contact with an agency or can be accounted for by other changes in their lives.

As regards AA, there are additional measuring problems: first of all, the voluntary nature of AA membership – the only requirement is "an honest desire to stop drinking" (Alcoholics Anonymous 1994: iv) – indicates that the ones attending meetings are not only recognising their drinking problem but are motivated to change (DiClemente et al. 1999 are critical of this assumption). "Because of this self-selection it becomes impossible to know whether it is AA efficacy or member motivation that is being measured" (Bebbington 1976 in Le, Ingvarson & Page 1995). Then there is the "on and off the wagon"-phenomenon (Ludwig 1989: 51-52) that complicates research. Further problems for research include: member anonymity, lack of control groups, the confounding effects of other treatment programs, frequency of attendance, and the informal nature of the movement (Le, Ingvarson and Page 1995; Glaser and Ogborne 1982). Moreover: "Not only does each person respond to personal events in different ways, but what moves one person toward sobriety may not affect another at all" (Ludwig 1989: 71). In sum, from a scientific point of view: the effectiveness of AA has yet to be proven.

3. DISCUSSION

It is questionable whether AA outcomes can be measured at all. Self-reports of sobriety are clearly not sufficient, as Glaser and Ogborne (1982: 125) argue and suggest that studies into the efficacy of AA also need to consider "how involvement with the movement contributes to psychological growth and the development of social skills particularly among (e.g.) depressed and/or socially incompetent individuals" (Glaser and Ogborne 1982: 125). Moreover, as Leach argues: "the study of AA may need 'unprecedented standards of measurement not appropriate to other treatment programs'" (Leach 1973 in Le, Ingvarson and Page 1995).

What also make studies into the effectiveness of AA so difficult is that there is "no general agreement about the nature, cause, or treatment of alcoholism" (Ludwig 1989: 3).

What, for instance, is recovery? There is no accepted definition of recovery. Moreover, the "lack of an accepted definition of *recovery* contributes significantly to the variability of reported outcomes of addiction treatment" (Maddux & Desmond 1986 in White 2007: 229).

While definitions are often arbitrary and may change over time, there is also a need to clarify what we mean when we speak of recovery, White argues, for there is a stigma attached to severe alcohol and other drug problems that will not disappear "until the meaning of recovery is clarified, the prevalence of recovery across cultural communities is confirmed by scientists, and a large cadre of individuals and families in long-term recovery stand to offer themselves as living proof of the transformative power of recovery" (White 2007: 230).

The following definition has been proposed: "Recovery from substance dependence is a voluntarily maintained lifestyle characterized by sobriety, personal health, and citizenship" (The Betty Ford Institute Consensus Panel 2007: 222). Sobriety here means abstinence, stable sobriety is considered to be achieved after 5 years; personal health means improved life quality (as defined and measured by World Health Organization standards) and citizenship means living with regard and respect for those around you (again as defined and measured by World Health Organization standards (The Betty Ford Institute Consensus Panel 2007).

It is doubtful that adhering to such bureaucratic standards will accomplish much. Moreover, it could very well be that the prevalent vague notions of recovery – "Recovery means change", Gorski (1989: 8) claims. "Recovery *is* and *demands* change. Recovery means that things have to be different than they were', Larsen (1985: 46) states and adds that "the core of the experience is that *enough is enough*" (Larsen 1985: 48). Nakken (1988: 89) holds that ' recovery is the process of becoming Self-centered" and that "Self-care, and a Self-relationship" is "the beginning of recovery" – are beneficial and serve a useful purpose for 'change' is a universal notion and commonly implies 'action' and 'better'.
It is the same purpose that Barack Obama's presidential campaign adhered to with its "Yes We Can"- slogan: We can do what? quite some commentators asked. They seem to have missed that the message was purposefully vague and thus allowed people to identify with whatever they wished 'but definitely something 'better').
In addition, it needs be noted that the search for a widely accepted definition of recovery is also a power struggle. There has been a remedicalisation of addiction treatment over the past two decades (McKeganey 2007 in Yates and Malloch 2010) and this substitute prescribing is fought against by advocates of "largely non-medical and, often, fiercely anti-treatment" (Yates and Malloch 2010) interventions.

In sum: that 'recovery' remains for many involved in mainstream specialist treatment a controversial area of addiction treatment (Day et al. 2005) has very probably to do with "our cultural and historical understanding of addiction and its consistent medicalisation over two centuries" (Yates and Malloch 2010). However,

The notion of calling a halt to a pattern of futile and self-destructive behaviour, of coming to an understanding of what drives that behaviour and changing it, overcoming it, is hundreds of years old. Traditionally, we have called it 'recovery' although, for many, the term 'discovery' may be more apposite (Yates and Malloch 2010)

Reviews of the available literature lead to the conclusion that the efficacy of AA has not been proven and that it "has not been demonstrated to be effective beyond what might

9

be expected by chance" (Glaser and Ogborne 1982:) yet as Glaser and Ogborne, when confronted with what AA members who often say, 'Of course AA works, we all know that', state: "To cut through an often endless and frequently acrimonious debate, let us say straightaway that we agree in general with such an assertion" (Glaser and Ogborne 1982:). Yet how can one say that when there isn't sufficient evidence of proof?

The fact that a cause-and-effect approach cannot prove whether AA works might indicate that the methodology used is probably not the most suitable to explain, and make sense of, the complexities of human behaviour not least because of too many variables. In addition, it is difficult to see how a causal approach could explain natural remission or spontaneous recovery.

What factors could indicate that AA is effective? There is, for instance, "a whole tradition of sociological studies of the actual functioning of AA, for the most part sympathetic" (Room, 1983: 77). There is also the fact that a spiritual approach works for some - Galanter et al. (2007) have identified "a number of studies on substance abusers' spiritual orientation whose findings reflect a positive relationship to recovery". Moreover, AA "has more than 2 million members in 100,000 groups scattered across 150 countries" (Adams 2009: 1) – on the other hand, one may also wonder why only about 5 to 10 percent of alcoholics in the US make use of it (Ludwig 1989: 67) – and there are statements like the one by Peck: "When I was in psychiatry training, back some thirty years ago, psychiatrists already knew that Alcoholics Anonymous had a much better track record in working with alcoholics than we psychiatrists had" (Peck 1993: 139). In addition, there are many recovered alcoholics who attribute their sobriety to AA (Zocker 1989; Robertson 1989).

Many personal testimonies (Wholey 1984; Ludwig 1989: 70-71, 79-81, 84-88) however show that stopping to drink is often not directly related to treatment but happens unexpectedly and strikes the one experiencing it as a miracle (what treatment may provide is to maintain the motivational batteries for *lasting* recovery). In the words of Ludwig (1989: 83-84):

The point is that as long as logical explanations or scientific theories fail to account for these extraordinary, spiritual experiences, assuming these reports of subsequent recovery to be true, then alcoholism may be more properly regarded as a "disease of the soul" than as a biological, behavioral, or social disorder, presumed to be caused and eventually cured by natural means. The question, simply put, is how to make scientific or clinical sense out of these claims without impugning the integrity of the individuals involved or regarding them as misguided or deluded.

Given that there is also "a substantial amount of spontaneous remission of drinking problems" (Roizen et al. 1978 cited in Room, 1983: 64), it is difficult to see how this can be accomplished. To paraphrase Shakespeare: there are more things in heaven and earth, than are dreamt of in our cause-and-effect philosophy. Moreover, as Watts (1973: 35) states:

We often say that you can only think of one thing at a time. The truth is that in looking at the world bit by bit we convince ourselves that it consists of separate things, and so give ourselves the problem of how these things are connected and how they cause and effect each other. The problem would never have arisen if we had been aware that it was just our way of looking at the world which had chopped it up into separate bits, things, events, causes, and effects. We do not see that the world is all of a piece ...

The classical AA-answer as to why one drinks ("Monday, Tuesday, Wednesday, Thursday, Friday, Saturday, Sunday") indicates that, in AA's view, to identify reasons for one's drinking is not of concern, what however matters is to act. "Fake it till you make it", as the AA-saying goes, *act yourself into a new way of thinking*, that is. In this AA differs from most therapeutic interventions (that try to make the addicts think into a new way of acting). Yet AA's action approach is not just a simple reversal of the more common approaches, it is also distinctly different in that it is full of contradictions and paradoxes and, instead of attempting to solve them, accepts them. For instance: "'Hitting bottom' is presumed to be a necessary step for recovery. even though being in dire straits, for all other illnesses, usually indicates a poor rather than favourable diagnosis" or "... the acceptance of personal weakness becomes the basis of strength" or "Once an alcoholic, always an alcoholic, as the saying goes. Even with cancer, the prognosis is not that grim" (Ludwig 1989: 3-4). What Creeley penned about life is equally true for addiction: "But it would be truly a fool who presumed any life to be simple consequence, or earned, or understood" (Clark 1993: 122).

AA is known as a simple programme for complicated people yet even these complicated people seem not to have been able to figure AA out. As Foster Wallace (1996: 349, 350) notes:

Nobody's ever been able to figure AA out, is another binding commonality. And the folks with serious time in AA are infuriating about questions starting with How. You ask the scary old guys How AA Works and they smile their chilly smiles and say Just Fine. It just works, is all; end of story

The claim that – despite the lack of cause-and-effect evidence – AA works (for the ones who work the programme, that is) is not only based on the personal experience of many (including my own) but also on the phenomenon that many things in life do work contrary to human logic (much of our created reality is based on mathematical models that work well despite claims by mathematicians that their basics are fundamentally flawed – Enzensberger 2009: 66). Furthermore, the AA-principles express centuries-old human wisdom; the generally non-doctrinaire approach (as an AA-slogan goes: "Take what you need and leave the rest" – Wakefield 1995: 8) is helpful and attractive; group affiliation (to identify with, and help, others) is a basic human need; "to act oneself into a new way of thinking" doesn't bother with the question why one drinks but shows how (h = honesty, o = openeness, w = willingness) to practically go about changing one's behaviour; and the Serenity Prayer

(God) grant me the serenity
to accept the things I cannot change,
the courage to change the things I can,
and the wisdom to know the difference

is presumably one of the better prescriptions for a sober and balanced life, "even for those who have trouble accepting the notion of a Higher Power" (Ludwig 1989: 134). As Ludwig (1989: 134) states "With this orientation to life, intoxication is unnecessary."

4. CONCLUSION

Since, there seem to be as many interpretations of AA as there are AA members and since it cannot be known how AA is individually practised, it is questionable whether AA allows for an assessment that meets scientific criteria. Yet despite the lack of scientific evidence, many believe – based on personal experience – that AA works. That these believers are all brainwashed seems unlikely (and would be difficult to prove) yet even if they were, the fact that they were drinking before joining AA and then stopped might indicate that their sobriety has something to do with AA.

Cause-and-effect methodologies seem not suited to explain the complexity of addiction and addiction treatment for they appear not able to make sense of the contradictions and paradoxes that are part of human behaviour. Moreover, they can't measure core factors such as motivation or belief that are crucial for any recovery. This failure also suggests that AA's *act yourself into a new way of thinking* might be preferable to treatment based on identifying causes and symptoms.

Future research and treatment need to find ways to address "the non-logical aspects" (the miracles, contradictions and paradoxes) of addiction and to adapt, complement, and possibly rethink, the cause-and-effect methodology.

5. REFERENCES

Adams, A.J. (2009) *Undrunk: A Skeptic's Guide to AA*, Center City: Hazelden.

Alcoholics Anonymous (1984) *"Pass it on". The story of Bill Wilson and how the A.A. message reacher the world,* New York: Alcoholics Anonymous World Services, Inc.

Alcoholics Anonymous (1994) *The Big Book: The Story of How Many Thousands of Men and Women Have Recovered from Alcoholism*, New York: Alcoholics Anonymous World Services, Inc.

Alcoholics Anonymous (1989) *Twelve Steps and Twelve Traditions*, New York: Alcoholics Anonymous World Services, Inc.

Ameisen, Olivier (2009) *Das Ende meiner Sucht (The End of My Addiction)*, München: Antje Kunstmann.

Bufe, Ch. (1998) *AA: Cult or Cure?*, Tucson: See Sharp Press; http://www.morerevealed.com/library/mr/newmr_0.jsp; accessed 12 March 2010.

Carey, B. (2008) 'The Evidence Gap Drug Rehabilitation or Revolving Door', *The New York Times*, p. D1 of the New York Edition; http://www.nytimes.com/2008/12/23/health/23reha.html?_r=3&scp=1&sq=drug%20reh abilitation&st=cse; accessed on 4 March 2010.

Clark, T. (1993) *Robert Creeley and the Genius of the American Common Place,* New York: New Directions.

Culter, R. and Fishbain, D. (2005) 'Are alcoholism treatments effective? The Project MATCH data' in *BMC Public Health,* http://www.biomedcentral.com/1471-2458/5/75; accessed 17 March 2010.

Day, E., Gaston, R., Furlong, E., Murali, V. & Coppello, A. (2005) 'United Kingdom substance misuse treatment workers' attitudes toward 12-step self-help groups' in *Journal of Substance Abuse Treatment*, 29: 321-327.

DiClemente, C.D., Bellino, L.E., Neavins, T.M. (1999) 'Motivation for Change and Alcoholism Treatment' in *Alcohol Research & Health*, Spring, http://findarticles.com/p/articles/mi_m0CXH/is_2_23/ai_59246571/?tag=content;col1; accessed 27 April 2010.

Enquist, P. O. (2009) *Ein anderes Leben (Another Life)*, München: Carl Hanser.

Enzensberger, H.M. (2009) *Fortuna und Kalkül. Zwei mathematische Belustigungen (Fortune and Calculus. Two mathematical amusements)*, Frankfurt am Main: Suhrkamp

Fletcher, A.M. (2001) *Sober for Good*, New York: Houghton Mifflin Company.

Foster Wallace, D. (1995) 'An Interval' in *The New Yorker*, 30 January; http://www.newyorker.com/archive/1995/01/30/1995_01_30_080_TNY_CARDS_0003 69136; accessed 8 March 2010.

Foster Wallace, D. (1996) *Infinite Jest*, Boston: Little, Brown and Company.

Franey, C., Ashton, M. (2002) 'The Grand design lessons from DATOS' in *Drug and Alcohol Findings*, 7: 4-19.

Fromm, E. (1979) *Sigmund Freuds Psychoanalyse - Grösse und Grenzen (Greatness and Limitations on Freud's Thought)*, Stuttgart: Deutsche Verlagsanstalt.

Galanter, M., Dermatis, H., Bunt, G., Williams, C., Trujillo, M., Steinke, P. (2007) 'Assessment of spirituality and its relevance to addiction treatment' in *Journal of Substance Abuse Treatment*, 33 (3): 257-264.

Glaser, F. B.; Ogborne, A.C. (1982) 'Does A.A. Really Work?' in *British Journal of Addiction*, 77: 123-129.

Goethals, I., Broekaert, E. and Yates, R. (forthcoming) 'A religion too far: On the hidden ideology of a social therapeutic belief system', (unpublished MS. submitted to *Mental Health and Substance Misuse*).

Gorski, T.T. (1989) *Passages Through Recovery*, Center City: Hazelden.

Jacques T. (1991) *De l'alcoholisme à la paix et à la sérénité (From alcoholism to peace and serenity)*, Cap-Saint-Ignace, Québec: Bibliothèque Québécoise.

James, W. (1994) *The Variety of Religious Experience,* New York: Random House.

Kurtz, E. (1991) *Not-God. A History of Alcoholics Anonymous*, Center City: Hazelden Pittman Archives Press.

Kurtz, E. (2004) 'Alcoholics Anonymous and the disease concept of alcoholism' in *Alcoholism Treatment Quarterly,* 20 (3/4): 107-130, http://www.bhrm.org/papers/AAand%20DiseaseConcept.pdf; accessed 27 April 2010.

Larsen, E. (1985) *Stage II Recovery. Life beyond addiction*, New York: HarperSanFrancisco.

Le, Ch., Ingvarson, E.P., Page, R.C. (1995) 'Alcoholics Anonymous and the Counseling Profession: Philosophies in conflict' in *Journal of Counseling & Development,* 7 January: 603; http://www.unhooked.com/sep/aacouns.htm, accessed 16 March 2010.

Ludwig, A.M. (1989) *Understanding the Alcoholic's Mind*, New York: Oxford University Press.

Maher, J.M, Briggs, D. (eds.) (1990) *An Open Life. Joseph Campbell in conversation with Michael Toms*, New York: Harper & Row, Publishers.

Miller, W. R., Rollnick, S., (2009) 'Ten Things that Motivational Interviewing Is Not' in *Behavioural and Cognitive Psychotherapy*, 37:129–140.

Nakken, C. (1988) *The Addictive Personality: Roots, Rituals, and Recovery*, Center City: Hazelden.

Peck, S. M. (1993) *Further along the road less traveled*, New York: Simon & Schuster.

Peele, S. (1995) *Diseasing of America: How we allowed recovery zealots and the treatment industry to convince us we are out of control,* Lexington MA/San Francisco: Lexington Books/Jossey-Bass; http://www.peele.net/lib/diseasing3.html, accessed 2 March 2010.

Peele, S. (1998) 'Introduction to to Charles Bufe's "AA: Cult or Cure"', http://www.peele.net/lib/bufe.html; accessed 12 March 2010.

Peele, S. (1998a) 'All Wet' in *The Sciences*, March/April: 17-21; http://peele.net/lib/allwet.html; accessed 16 March 2010.

Project MATCH Research Group (1993) 'Project MATCH: Rationale and methods for a multisite clinical trial matching patients to alcoholism treatment' in *Alcoholism: Clinical and Experimental Research*, 17: 1130-1145.

Robertson, N. (1989) *Die Anonymen Alkoholiker. Der erfolgreiche Weg aus der Sucht (The title of the English original is "Getting Better')*. München: Droemer Knaur.

Room, R. (1983) 'Sociology and the Disease Concept of Alcoholism' in *Research Advances in Alcohol and Drug Problems*, 7, New York and London Plenum Press.

Rudy, D.R., Greil, A.L. (1988) 'Is Alcoholics Anonymous a Religious Organization?: Meditations on Marginality' in *Sociological Analysis*, 50, Abstract, http://www.jstor.org/pss/3710917; accessed 13 April 2010.

Sheed, W. (1995) *In Love with Daylight. A Memoir of Recovery*. New York. Simon & Schuster.

The Betty Ford Institute Consensus Panel (2007) 'What is recovery? A working definition from the Betty Ford Institute' in *Journal of Substance Abuse Treatment*, 33 (3): 221–228.

This is A.A. (1984) 'An introduction to the A.A. recovery program'. http://www.aa.org/pdf/products/p-1_thisisaa1.pdf; accessed 22 February 2010.

Trimpey, J. (1997) 'Alcoholics Anonymous: Of Course It's a Cult!' in *The Journal of Rational Recovery,* 9 (5), May-June, 1997; http://www.positiveatheism.org/rw/ofcourse.htm, accessed 1 March 2010.

Vaillant, G. E. (1983) *Natural History of Alcoholism,* Cambridge MA, Harvard University Press.

Velasquez, M.M., DiClemente, C.D., Addy, R.C. (2000) 'Generalizability of Project Match: a comparison of clients enrolled to those not enrolled in the study at one aftercare site' in *Drug and Alcohol Dependence*, 59: 177–182.

Wakefield, D. (1995) *Expect a Miracle*, New York: HarperSanFrancisco.

Watts, A. (1973) *The book on the taboo against knowing who you are*, New York: Abacus.

West, J.W. (1997) *The Betty Ford Center Book of Answers,* New York: Pocket Books.

White, W. L. (2007) 'Addiction recovery: Its definition and conceptual boundaries' in *Journal of Substance Abuse Treatment*, 33 (3): 229–241.

White, W. L. (2007a) 'Recovery as a Heroic Journey'; http://www.facesandvoicesofrecovery.org/pdf/White/recovery_as_heroic_journey.pdf; accessed 8 March 2010.

Wholey, D. (1984) *The Courage to Change*, New York: Warner Books.

Yates, R. (1997) *A Guide to Developing Services for Alcohol and Drug Misusers*, Edinburgh: The Scottish Office.

Yates, R., Malloch, M. (2010) 'The road less travelled? a short history of addiction recovery' in Yates, R. and Malloch, M. (eds.) *Tackling Addiction: Pathways to Recovery*, London: Jessica Kingsley Publishers, pp. 15-31.

Zocker, H. (1989) betrifft: *Anonyme Alkoholiker: Selbsthilfe gegen die Sucht (concerns: Alcoholics Anonymous: Self-help against addiction)*, München: Beck

24 Magazine (1976) 'Gresham's Law & Alcoholics Anonymous'; http://www.barefootsworld.net/aagreshamslaw.html; accessed 7 March 2010

———

6. APPENDIX

THE TWELVE STEPS

1. We admitted we were powerless over alcohol - that our lives had become unmanageable.

2. Came to believe that a power greater than ourselves could restore us to sanity.

3. Made a decision to turn our will and our lives over to the care of God as we understood Him.

4. Made a searching and fearless moral inventory of ourselves.

5. Admitted to God, to ourselves, and to another human being the exact nature of our wrongs.

6. Were entirely ready to have God remove all these defects of character.

7. Humbly asked Him to remove our shortcomings.

8. Made a list of all persons we had harmed, and became willing to make amends to them all.

9. Made direct amends to such people wherever possible, except when to do so would injure them or others.

10. Continued to take personal inventory and when we were wrong, promptlym admitted it.

11. Sought though prayer and meditation to improve our conscious contact with God as we understood Him, praying only for knowledge of His will for us and the power to carry that out.

12. Having had a spiritual awakening as the result of these steps, we tried to carry this message to alcoholics and to practice these principles in all our affairs.

THE TWELVE TRADITIONS

1. Our common welfare should come first; personal recovery depends upon A.A. unity.

2. For our group purpose there is but one ultimate authority - a loving God as He may express Himself in our group conscience. Our leaders are but trusted servants; they do not govern.

3. The only requirement for A.A. membership is a desire to stop drinking.

4. Each group should be autonomous except in matters affecting other groups or A.A. as a whole.

5. Each group has but one primary purpose - to carry its message to the alcoholic who still suffers.

6. An A.A. group ought never endorse, finance or lend the A.A. name to any related facility or outside enterprise, lest problems of money, property and prestige divert us from our primary purpose.

7. Every A.A. group ought to be fully self-supporting, declining outside contributions.

8. Alcoholics Anonymous should remain forever non-professional, but our service

centers may employ special workers.

9. A.A., as such, ought never be organized; but we may create service boards or committees directly responsible to those they serve.

10. Alcoholics Anonymous has no opinion on outside issues; hence the A.A. name ought never be drawn into public controversy.

11. Our public relations policy is based on attraction rather than promotion; we need always maintain personal anonymity at the level of press, radio and films.

12. Anonymity is the spiritual foundation of all our traditions, ever reminding us to place principles before personalities.

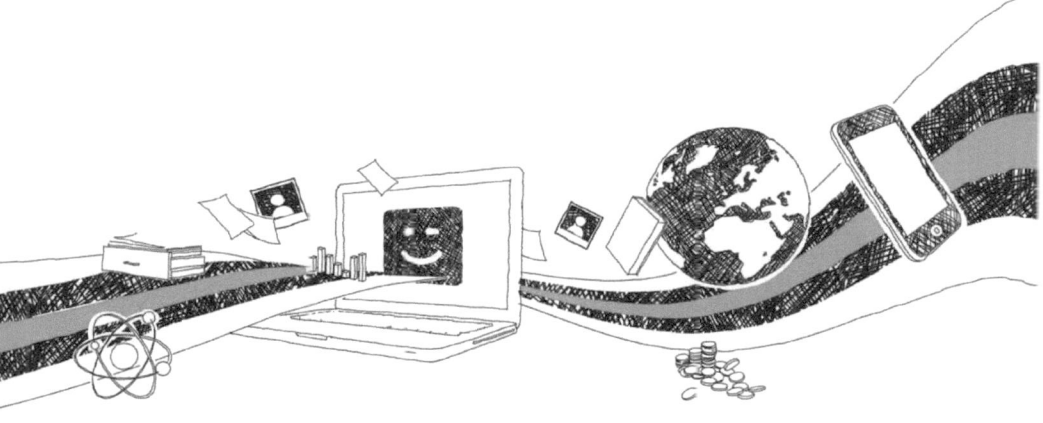